KETO DIET COOKBOOK

FOR BEGINNERS:

SMOOTHIES AND DRINK RECIPES

Quick, Easy and Delicious Recipes
for healthy living while keeping
your weight under control

Amanda Grant

Copyright © 2021 by Amanda Grant

Legal Disclaimer

The information contained in this book and its contents is not designed to replace any form of medical or professional advice; and is not meant to replace the need for independent medical, financial, legal, or other professional advice or service that may require. The content and information in this book have been provided for educational and entertainment purposes only.

The content and information contained in this book have been compiled from sources deemed reliable, and they are accurate to the best of the Author's knowledge, information and belief.

However, the Author cannot guarantee its accuracy and validity and therefore cannot be held liable for any errors and/or omissions.

Further, changes are periodically made to this book as needed. Where appropriate and/or necessary, you must consult a professional (including but not limited to your doctor, attorney, financial advisor, or other such professional) before using any of the suggested remedies, techniques, and/or information in this book.

Upon using this book's contents and information, you agree to hold harmless the Author from any damaged, costs and expenses, including any legal fees potentially resulting from the application of any of the information in this book. This disclaimer applies to any loss, damages, or injury caused by the use and application of this book's content, whether directly and indirectly, whether for breach of contract, tort, negligence, personal injury, criminal intent, or under any other circumstances.

You agree to accept all risks of using the information presented in this book. You agree that by continuing to read this book, where appropriate and/or necessary, you shall consult a professional (including but not limited to your doctor, attorney, financial advisor, or other such professional) before remedies, techniques, and/or information in this book.

TABLE OF CONTENTS

Coffee With Cream...8

Keto Coffee...9

Vegan Keto Golden Milk 10

Keto Creamy Chocolate Smoothie 11

Keto Pumpkin Pie Spice Latte 12

Blueberry Banana Bread Smoothie 14

Blackberry Chocolate Shake 15

Dairy-Free Dark Chocolate Shake 16

Keto Meal Replacement Shake.........................18

Keto Iced Coffee 19

Low-Carb Ginger Smoothie 20

Whipped Dairy-Free Low-Carb Dalgona Coffee 21

Keto Eggnog 23

Iced Tea 25

Flavored Water 26

Butter Coffee 27

Keto Hot Chocolate 28

Dairy-Free Keto Latte 29

Low-Carb Vegan Vanilla Protein Shake.................30

Electrolyte Elixir 31

Keto Chai Latte 32

Sugar-Free Mulled Wine 33

Co-Keto (Puerto Rican Coconut Eggnog) 34

Cinnamon Coffee 36

Sugar-Free Caramel Brulee Latte 37

Pumpkin Spice Latte Milkshakes 38

Keto Russian Coffee 40

Creamy Matcha Latte 41

Keto Avocado Smoothie 42

Avocado Mint Green Keto Smoothie 43

Keto Skinny Margaritas 44

Iced Keto Matcha Green Tea Latte 45

Spiced Gingerbread Coffee 46

Coconut Milk Strawberry Smoothie 47

Peanut Butter Chocolate Keto Milkshake 48

Sugar-Free Fresh Squeezed Lemonade 49

Cucumber Mint Water 50

Caramel Apple Drink 51

Keto Frosty Chocolate Shake 53

Strawberry Avocado Smoothie 54

Almond Berry Mini Cheesecake Smoothies 55

Hemp Milk And Nut Milk 57

Gut Healing Bone Broth Latte 59

Creamy Cocoa Coconut Low Carb Shake 61

Low Carb Dark Chocolate Protein Smoothie 62

Mint Chocolate Green Smoothie 63

Low Carb Raspberry Cheesecake Shake 64

Watermelon Smoothie 65

Low-Carb Blueberry Smoothie 66

Pumpkin Low Carb Smoothie With Salted Caramel 67

McKeto Strawberry Milkshake 68

Keto Blueberry Cheesecake Smoothie 69

Keto Tropical Smoothie 70

Keto Kale & Coconut Shake 71

Savory Cucumber Herb Sangria 72

Sparkling Raspberry Limeade Mocktail 74

Bailey's Irish Cream 75

Low Carb Coffee Milkshake 76

Sugar-Free Strawberry Limeade 77

Low-Carb Keto Shamrock Shake 78

Keto Smoothie With Almond Milk 79

Sparkling Grapefruit Frosé 80

Banana Oat Breakfast Smoothie 81

Keto Mexican Chocolate Eggnog 82

Keto Cranberry Hibiscus Margarita 84

Keto Frozen Blackberry Lemonade 86

Triple Berry Cheesecake Smoothie 87

ServMaple Almond 88

Dairy Free Chocolate Pecan Keto Shake 89

Strawberry Colada Milkshake 90

Keto Frozen Hot Chocolate 91

Dairy-Free Keto Iced Latte 93

Sugar-Free Hibiscus Lemonade 94

Low Carb 7Up **95**

Low Carb German Chocolate Fat Bomb Hot Chocolate... **96**

Low Carb German Gingerbread Hot Chocolate **97**

Coconut Pumpkin Steamer.................................... **99**

Low Carb Margarita Mix **100**

Low Carb Electrolyte Water **101**

Low Carb Pumpkin Spice Mocha **102**

Kombucha Sangria... **103**

Pumpkin Spice Hot Buttered Rum....................... **104**

Tart Cherry Lemon Drop **106**

Orange Creamsicle Mimosas **108**

KETO DIET: DRINK AND SMOOTHIES

Coffee With Cream

Servings: 1 | Time: 5 mins | Difficulty: Easy

INGREDIENTS:

1. 1/4 Cup Heavy Whipping Cream
2. 2 Tbsps. Nuts, Crushed (Optional)
3. 3/4 Cup Brewed Coffee

DIRECTIONS:

1. Brew your coffee according to your preference.
2. Slightly heat the cream in a pan and stir till it becomes frothy.
3. Take a cup and mix the warm cream and coffee in it.
4. Serve hot with crushed nuts on top or as it is.

Nutrients per serving: Calories: 203 kcal | Fat: 21g | Carbohydrates: 2g | Protein: 2g | Fiber: 0g

Keto Coffee

Servings: 2 | Time: 5 mins | Difficulty: Easy

INGREDIENTS:

- ➢ 2 Tbsps. Coconut Oil Or MCT Oil
- ➢ 2 Tbsps. Butter, Unsalted (Grass-Fed)
- ➢ 2 Cups Brewed Coffee
- ➢ 1 Tsp. Vanilla Extract (Optional)
- ➢ 1 Tbsp. Heavy Whipping Cream (Optional)

DIRECTIONS:

1. Brew your coffee according to your preference.
2. Blend the coffee with unsalted butter, coconut or MCT oil, vanilla extract, and whipping cream if you want, in a blender for about a minute or until it becomes frothy.
3. Pour out the keto coffee in your favorite mugs and enjoy.

Nutrients per serving: Calories: 260 kcal | Fat: 27.7g | Carbohydrates: 1.05g | Protein: 1.08g | Fiber: 0g

Vegan Keto Golden Milk

Servings: 1 | Time: 5 mins | Difficulty: Easy

INGREDIENTS:

- ➢ 2 Tsps. Ginger, Fresh & Peeled
- ➢ 2 Tbsps. MCT Oil
- ➢ 1 & 1/2 Cup Almond Milk, Unsweetened
- ➢ 2 Tsps. Erythritol
- ➢ 1/4 Tsp. Cinnamon, Ground
- ➢ 2 Ice Cubes
- ➢ 3/4 Tsp. Turmeric Powder
- ➢ 1/4 Tsp. Vanilla Extract
- ➢ Sea Salt, To Taste

DIRECTIONS:

1. Combine all the INGREDIENTS:in a blender and mix for about a quarter or half a minute.

2. For the strong taste of turmeric and ginger, blend longer.

3. Decant into the glass or mug and sprinkle powdered cinnamon on top before serving.

Nutrients per serving: Calories: 303 kcal | Fat: 31.1g | Carbohydrates: 2.7g | Protein: 2.1g | Fiber: 2g

Keto Creamy Chocolate Smoothie

Servings: 2 | Time: 10 mins | Difficulty: Easy

INGREDIENTS:

- ➢ 1 Tbsp. Almond Butter
- ➢ 1 Tsp. Coconut Oil
- ➢ 1/2 Avocado
- ➢ 1 Tbsp. Flax Meal
- ➢ 1 & 1/4 Cups Almond Milk, Unsweetened
- ➢ 1 Tbsp. Cocoa Powder, Unsweetened
- ➢ 1/4 Cup Heavy Whipping Cream
- ➢ Liquid Stevia, To Taste

DIRECTIONS:

1. Combine all the INGREDIENTS:in a blender and mix until a smooth consistency is attained.

2. Decant into the serving glass and top with cocoa powdered and whipped cream if you want.

Nutrients per serving: Calories: 593.3 kcal | Fat: 55.7g | Carbohydrates: 7.7g | Protein: 10.6g | Fiber: 11.7g

Keto Pumpkin Pie Spice Latte

Servings: 3 | Time: 10 mins | Difficulty: Easy

INGREDIENTS:

- ➢ 2 Tbsps. Butter
- ➢ 1/2 Tsp. Cinnamon, Powdered
- ➢ 1 Cup Coconut Milk
- ➢ 2 Cups Brewed Coffee
- ➢ 2 Tsps. Pumpkin Pie Spice
- ➢ 1/4 Cup Pumpkin Puree
- ➢ 1 Tsp. Vanilla Extract
- ➢ 2 Tbsps. Heavy Whipping Cream
- ➢ 15 Drops Liquid Stevia

DIRECTIONS:

1. Pour the coconut milk, butter, pumpkin puree, and spices into a small saucepan and heat over a medium-low flame.
2. Once the mixture starts to bubble, add the coffee, and mix well.
3. Remove from the heat and add the whipped cream and liquid Stevia. Mix well to blend the contents until frothy.

4. Decant in the serving mug and a dollop of whipped cream on top.

Blueberry Banana Bread Smoothie

Servings: 2 | Time: 10 mins | Difficulty: Easy

INGREDIENTS:

- 1/4 Cup Blueberries
- 2 Tbsps. MCT Oil
- 2 1 & 1/2 Tsps. Banana Extract
- Cups Vanilla Coconut Milk, Unsweetened
- 1 Tbsp. Chia Seeds
- 3 Tbsps. Golden Flaxseed Meal
- 10 Drop Liquid Stevia
- 1/4 Tsp. Xanthan Gum

DIRECTIONS:

1. Combine all the INGREDIENTS:in a blender and let it sit for a few minutes to allow the chia and flax seeds to soak some moisture.

2. Then blend for a minute or two until a smooth consistency is attained.

3. Serve in the glasses and enjoy.

Nutrients per serving: Calories: 270 kcal | Fat: 23.31g | Carbohydrates: 4.66g | Protein: 3.13g | Fiber: 5.65g

Blackberry Chocolate Shake

Servings: 2 | Time: 5 mins | Difficulty: Easy

INGREDIENTS:

- 1/4 Cup Blackberries
- 2 Tbsps. MCT Oil
- 1 Cup Coconut Milk, Unsweetened
- 1/4 Tsp. Xanthan Gum
- 2 Tbsps. Cocoa Powder
- 12 Drops Liquid Stevia
- 7 Ice Cubes

DIRECTIONS:

1. Combine all the **INGREDIENTS:**in a blender and blend for a minute or two until a smooth consistency is attained.

2. Serve in the glasses and enjoy.

Nutrients per serving: Calories: 346 kcal | Fat: 34.17g | Carbohydrates: 4.8g | Protein: 2.62g | Fiber: 7.4g

Dairy-Free Dark Chocolate Shake

Servings: 2 | Time: 5 mins | Difficulty: Easy

INGREDIENTS:

- ➢ 1/2 Avocado
- ➢ 1/2 Cup Coconut Cream, Chilled
- ➢ 2 Tbsps. Hulled Hemp Seeds
- ➢ 2 Tbsps. Dark Chocolate (Low Carb)
- ➢ 1/2 Cup Almond Milk
- ➢ 1 Tbsp. Cocoa Powder
- ➢ 2 Tbsps. Powdered Erythritol, To Taste
- ➢ Flake Salt, To Taste
- ➢ 1 Cup Ice

DIRECTIONS:

1. Put the cocoa powder, hemp seeds, erythritol, and dark chocolate in a blender and mix until the chocolate is chopped.
2. Add the remaining **INGREDIENTS:**and blend for a minute or two until a smooth consistency is attained.
3. Pour in the serving glasses and enjoy.

<u>Nutrients per serving</u>: Calories: 349.35 kcal | Fat: 33.15g | Carbohydrates: 5.73g | Protein: 7.2g | Fiber: 6.1g

Keto Meal Replacement Shake

Servings: 2 | Time: 5 mins | Difficulty: Easy

INGREDIENTS:

➢ 1/2 Avocado

➢ 2 Tbsps. Almond Butter

➢ 1 Cup Almond Or Coconut Milk, Unsweetened

➢ 1/4 Tsp. Vanilla Extract

➢ 1/2 Tsp. Cinnamon, Powdered

➢ 2 Tbsps. Golden Flaxseed Meal

➢ 1/8 Tsp. Salt

➢ 2 Tbsp. Cocoa Powder

➢ 1/2 Cup Heavy Cream

➢ 15 Drops Liquid Stevia

➢ 8 Ice Cubes

DIRECTIONS:

1. Combine all the INGREDIENTS:in a blender and blend for a minute or two until a smooth consistency is attained.

2. Serve in the glasses and enjoy.

Keto Iced Coffee

Servings: 1 | Time: 5 mins | Difficulty: Easy

INGREDIENTS:

- ➢ 3 Tbsps. Heavy Cream
- ➢ 5 Drops Liquid Stevia
- ➢ 1 Cup Brewed Coffee
- ➢ 1/2 Tsp. Vanilla Extract (Optional)
- ➢ Ice Cubes, To Taste

DIRECTIONS:

1. Brew your coffee according to your preference and let it cool down to room temperature.

2. Combine the coffee with all the other INGREDIENTS:in a blender and blend for about a minute or until it becomes frothy.

3. Pour the iced coffee in your favorite mug and enjoy.

Nutrients per serving: Calories: 160 kcal | Fat: 16.1g | Carbohydrates: 1.5g | Protein: 1.6g | Fiber: 0g

Low-Carb Ginger Smoothie

Servings: 2 | Time: 5 mins | Difficulty: Easy

INGREDIENTS:

➢ 2 Tbsps. Spinach, Frozen

➢ 1/3 Cup Coconut Milk Or Cream, Unsweetened

➢ 2 Tsps. Ginger, Fresh & Grated

➢ 2 Tbsps. Lime Juice, Divided

➢ 2/3 Cup Water

For Garnishing

➢ 1/2 Tsp. Fresh Ginger, Grated

DIRECTIONS:

1. Combine all the **INGREDIENTS:** in a blender and adjust the lime juice amount as per your taste.

2. Blend the mixture for a minute or until a smooth consistency is attained.

3. Serve with grated ginger on top.

Nutrients per serving: Calories: 83 kcal | Fat: 8g | Carbohydrates: 3g | Protein: 1g | Fiber: 1g

Whipped Dairy-Free Low-Carb Dalgona Coffee

Servings: 2 | Time: 5 mins | Difficulty: Easy

INGREDIENTS:

- 2 Tbsps. Water, Hot
- 1 & 1/2 Cups Coconut Or Almond Milk, Unsweetened
- 1 & 1/2 Tbsps. Erythritol
- 1 & 1/2 Tbsps. Espresso Instant Coffee Powder
- 1/2 Cup Ice Cubes
- 1 Tsp. Vanilla Extract (Optional)

DIRECTIONS:

1. Take a narrow glass and combine the coffee powder, hot water, and erythritol in it and blend them well with an immersion blender for about 3 minutes or till the mixture becomes creamy and light in color.

2. Take two glasses, fill two-third of them with ice and then pour the almond or coconut milk in it along with vanilla extract if you want. Mix them well.

3. Put the spoonful of the creamy coffee mixture on the top of each glass and stir before serving.

Nutrients per serving: Calories: 40 kcal | Fat: 2g | Carbohydrates: 1g | Protein: 1g | Fiber: 1g

Keto Eggnog

Servings: 4 | Time: 10 mins | Difficulty: Easy

INGREDIENTS:

- ➢ 1/4 Cup Orange Juice
- ➢ 2 Egg Yolks
- ➢ 1/2 Tbsp. Orange Zest
- ➢ 1/4 Tbsp. Vanilla
- ➢ 1/2 Tsp. Erythritol, Powdered
- ➢ 1/8 Tsp. Nutmeg, Ground
- ➢ 1 Cup Heavy Whipping Cream
- ➢ 4 Tbsps. Bourbon Or Brandy (Optional)

DIRECTIONS:

1. Combine egg yolks, vanilla extract, and erythritol in a deep bowl and whisk the mixture well until it becomes fluffy.

2. Add in the orange juice, orange zest, and whipping cream. Mix well until a smooth consistency is attained.

3. Pour the eggnog n the serving glasses and refrigerate for about 15 minutes.

4. Finally, serve with a sprinkle of nutmeg on top.

<u>Nutrients per serving:</u> Calories: 249 kcal | Fat: 24g | Carbohydrates: 6g | Protein: 3g | Fiber: 1g

Iced Tea

Servings: 2 | Time: 2 hrs. & 10 mins | Difficulty: Easy

INGREDIENTS:

- ➢ 1 Tea Bag
- ➢ 2 Cups Cold Water
- ➢ 1 Cup Ice Cubes
- ➢ 1/3 Cup Sliced Lemon or Fresh Mint Leaves

DIRECTIONS:

1. Put the teabag and lemon slices or mint leaves in a cup of cold water in a pitcher and put in the refrigerator for an hour or two.

2. Take the tea bag, and lemon slices or mint leaves out of the water. Substitute them with new ones if you want.

3. Pour in another cup of water and ice cubes in the pitcher and serve.

Nutrients per serving: Calories: 0 kcal | Fat: 0g | Carbohydrates: 0g | Protein: 0g | Fiber: 0g

Flavored Water

Servings: 4 | Time: 5 mins | Difficulty: Easy

INGREDIENTS:

- ➢ 2 Cups Ice Cubes
- ➢ Flavoring, e.g., Fresh Mint Or Raspberries, Or Sliced Cucumber
- ➢ 4 Cups Cold Water

DIRECTIONS:

1. Take a pitcher and add cold water along with flavorings in it.
2. Refrigerate it for about 30 minutes and then serve.

Nutrients per serving: Calories: 0 kcal | Fat: 0g | Carbohydrates: 0g | Protein: 0g | Fiber: 0g

Butter Coffee

Servings: 1 | Time: 5 mins | Difficulty: Easy

INGREDIENTS:

➢ 2 Tbsps. Butter, Unsalted

➢ 1 Tbsp. Coconut Or MCT Oil

➢ 1 Cup Freshly Brewed Coffee, Hot

DIRECTIONS:

1. Brew your coffee according to your preference, and let it cool down a bit.

2. Combine the coffee with all the other **INGREDIENTS:**in a blender and blend for about a minute or until it becomes frothy.

3. Pour the butter coffee in your favorite mug and enjoy.

Nutrients per serving: Calories: 0 kcal | Fat: 37g | Carbohydrates: 0g | Protein: 1g | Fiber: 0g

Keto Hot Chocolate

Servings: 1 | Time: 5 mins | Difficulty: Easy

INGREDIENTS:

➢ Cup Boiling Water

➢ & 1/2 Tsps. Powdered Erythritol

➢ Tbsps. Butter, Unsalted

➢ 1/4 Tsp. Vanilla Extract

➢ Tbsp. Cocoa Powder

DIRECTIONS:

1. Combine all the **INGREDIENTS:**in a full-sized mug and blend well with an immersion blender until it becomes frothy.

2. Serve hot and enjoy.

Nutrients per serving: Calories: 216 kcal | Fat: 23g | Carbohydrates: 1g | Protein: 1g | Fiber: 2g

Dairy-Free Keto Latte

Servings: 2 | Time: 5 mins | Difficulty: Easy

INGREDIENTS:

➢ 1 & 1/2 Cups Boiling Water

➢ 2 Tbsps. Coconut Oil

➢ 1 Tsp. Ground Ginger Or Pumpkin Pie Spice

➢ 2 Eggs

➢ 1/8 Tsp. Vanilla Extract

DIRECTIONS:

1. Combine all the **INGREDIENTS:**in a blender and blend for a few seconds.

2. Do not let the eggs cook in the boiling water and serve instantly.

Nutrients per serving: Calories: 191 kcal | Fat: 18g | Carbohydrates: 1g | Protein: 6g | Fiber: 0g

Low-Carb Vegan Vanilla Protein Shake

Servings: 1 | Time: 10 mins | Difficulty: Easy

INGREDIENTS:

- ➢ 4 Tbsps. Pea Protein Powder, Unflavored
- ➢ 1/2 Cup Almond Milk, Unsweetened
- ➢ 2 Tbsps. Cauliflower Rice, Frozen
- ➢ 1 Tbsp. Almond Butter
- ➢ 1/2 Cup Coconut Milk
- ➢ 1 Tsp. Vanilla Extract
- ➢ 1/2 Tsp. Cinnamon, Ground

DIRECTIONS:

1. Combine all the INGREDIENTS:in a blender and blend the mixture for a minute or until a smooth consistency is attained.

2. Decant in a serving glass and enjoy.

Nutrients per serving: Calories: 449 kcal | Fat: 34g | Carbohydrates: 8g | Protein: 28g | Fiber: 4g

Electrolyte Elixir

Servings: 4 | Time: 1 min | Difficulty: Easy

INGREDIENTS:

- ➢ 1/2 Cup Lemon Juice, Fresh
- ➢ 1/2 Tsp. Magnesium
- ➢ 1 Tsp. Salt
- ➢ 8 Cups Water

DIRECTIONS:

1. Combine all the **INGREDIENTS:**in a pitcher and stir well.
2. Decant in serving glasses and enjoy.

Nutrients per serving: Calories: 7 kcal | Fat: 0.1g | Carbohydrates: 2g | Protein: 0.1g | Fiber: 0g

Keto Chai Latte

Servings: 2 | Time: 5 mins | Difficulty: Beginner

INGREDIENTS:

- ➢ 2 Cups Boiling Water
- ➢ 1/3 Cup Heavy Whipping Cream
- ➢ 1 Tbsp. Chai Tea

DIRECTIONS:

1. According to the package instructions, brew the tea in boiling water.

2. In a saucepan or microwave, heat the cream and pour it into the tea and serve.

Nutrients per serving: Calories: 133 kcal | Fat: 14g | Carbohydrates: 1g | Protein: 1g | Fiber: 0g

Sugar-Free Mulled Wine

Servings: 8 | Time: 15 mins | Difficulty: Beginner

INGREDIENTS:

- ➢ 2 Cinnamon Sticks
- ➢ 1 & 1/2 Tsps. Orange Zest, Dried
- ➢ 1 Star Anise
- ➢ 2 Tsps. Ginger, Dried
- ➢ 1 Tsp. Green Cardamom Seeds
- ➢ 3 Cups White Or Red Wine, With Or Without Alcohol
- ➢ 1 Tsp. Cloves
- ➢ 1 Tbsp. Vanilla Extract (Optional)

DIRECTIONS:

1. Combine all the **INGREDIENTS:**in a saucepan and simmer over medium-low flame for about 5-10 minutes. Do not bring to boil.

2. Remove from the heat and let the mixture sit overnight for a strong taste of spices.

3. Strain the wine and serve hot with snacks or nuts.

Nutrients per serving: Calories: 82 kcal | Fat: 0.1g | Carbohydrates: 3g | Protein: 0.1g | Fiber: 0g

Co-Keto (Puerto Rican Coconut Eggnog)

Servings: 2 | Time: 5 mins | Difficulty: Easy

INGREDIENTS:

- ➢ 3 & 1/3 Cups Coconut Cream
- ➢ 2 Cups Heavy Whipping Cream
- ➢ 4 Egg Yolks, Beaten
- ➢ 1 & 2/3 Cups Coconut Milk, Unsweetened
- ➢ 1 Cup Rum
- ➢ 1/2 Cup Warm Water
- ➢ 2 Tbsps. Coconut Oil
- ➢ 1 Tbsp. Vanilla Extract
- ➢ Stevia, To Taste
- ➢ 2 Tsps. Cinnamon, Ground
- ➢ 1/4 Tsp. Ginger, Ground
- ➢ 1/4 Tsp. Nutmeg, Ground
- ➢ 1/4 Tsp. Cloves, Ground

DIRECTIONS:

1. Heat the beaten egg yolks and whipping cream together in a double boiler, constantly stirring until a smooth consistency is attained and the temperature reaches 160°F.

2. Add the coconut oil and mix well until thick and smooth.

3. Pour this mixture into a blender and add all the other ingredients. Blend well and then transfer to the glass bottles and let chill.

Nutrients per serving: Calories: 563kcal | Fat: 56g| Carbohydrates: 7g | Protein: 7g| Fiber: 0g

Cinnamon Coffee

Servings: 1 | Time: 5 mins | Difficulty: Easy

INGREDIENTS:

➢ 1/2 Tsp. Brown Sugar

➢ 1/8 Tsp. Cinnamon, Powdered

➢ Whipped Cream (Optional)

➢ 1 Cup Coffee

DIRECTIONS:

1. According to the package instructions, brew the coffee.

2. Add the brown sugar and cinnamon powder to it and stir well.

3. Put a dollop of whipped cream on top if you want.

Nutrients per serving: Calories: 660 kcal | Fat: 60g | Carbohydrates: 7g | Protein: 13g | Fiber: 7g

Sugar-Free Caramel Brulee Latte

Servings: 2 | Time: 2 mins | Difficulty: Easy

INGREDIENTS:

➢ 2 Tbsps. Caramel Syrup

➢ 2 Cups Brewed Coffee

➢ 4 Tbsps. Coconut Milk Or Heavy Whipped Cream

DIRECTIONS:

1. Brew your coffee according to your preference and add one Tbsp. of caramel syrup and 2 Tbsps. of coconut milk or heavy cream in each cup.

2. Top with a dollop of whipped cream or caramel if you want and serve.

Nutrients per serving: Calories: 106 kcal | Fat: 11g | Carbohydrates: 1g | Protein: 1g |

Pumpkin Spice Latte Milkshakes

Servings: 3 | Time: 15 mins | Difficulty: Easy

INGREDIENTS:

➢ 1 Cup Keto Vanilla Ice Cream

➢ 1/3 Cup Almond Milk

➢ 1/3 Cup Water

➢ 2 Tbsps. Pumpkin Puree

➢ 1 & 1/2 Tsp. Instant Coffee

➢ 1 Tsp. Pumpkin Pie Spice

Coconut Whipped Cream:

➢ 2 Tbsps. Sugar (Low Carb)

➢ 1 & 3/4 Cups Coconut Milk

DIRECTIONS:

1. Put the coconut milk in the refrigerator overnight, take the thick cream off the milk top, and put it in a bowl. Save the milk for other recipes.

2. Whisk in the low carb sugar in the coconut cream until your desired consistency is attained.

3. Combine all the other INGREDIENTS:in a blender and blend for a few minutes until it becomes smooth.

4. Decant in your preferred glasses and top with coconut whipped cream.

Nutrients per serving (with 2 Tbsps. whipped coconut cream per shake): Calories: 364 kcal | Fat: 18.52g| Carbohydrates: 5.48g | Protein: 2.3g| Fiber: 1.83g

Keto Russian Coffee

Servings: 2 | Time: 2 mins | Difficulty: Easy

INGREDIENTS:

- ➢ 1/3 Cup Vanilla Vodka
- ➢ 4 Tbsps. Almond Milk, Unsweetened
- ➢ 2 Tbsps. Stevia
- ➢ 2 Cups Brewed Coffee

Milk Foam (Optional)

- ➢ 1/4 Cup Heavy Cream
- ➢ 2 Tbsps. French Vanilla Whipped Foam Topping (Sugar-Free)
- ➢ 1 Stick Of Cinnamon
- ➢ 1/4 Tsp. Vanilla Extract

DIRECTIONS:

1. Brew coffee according to your preference and divide it into two cups. Stir in half of the almond milk, Stevia, and vodka in each cup.
2. Put the milk foam on top if you want.
3. To make milk foam, combine all its **INGREDIENTS:**in a jar and mix well until the mixture becomes frothy. Microwave for 10 sec and then put a dollop on each serving.

Creamy Matcha Latte

Servings: 1 | Time: 6 mins | Difficulty: Easy

INGREDIENTS:

- ➢ 1/8 Tsp. Pink Sea Salt
- ➢ 1/3 Cup Almond Milk, Unsweetened
- ➢ 1 Tsp. Matcha Tea
- ➢ 2/3 Cup Coconut Milk
- ➢ Stevia, To Taste
- ➢ 4 Drops Vanilla Extract (Optional)

DIRECTIONS:

1. Take a saucepan and add both kinds of milk to it. Heat until it starts to bubble and add the remaining **INGREDIENTS:**to it.
2. Mix well and serve in separate cups.

Nutrients per serving: Calories: 255 kcal | Fat: 22.8g| Carbohydrates: 5.3g | Protein: 2.33g | Fiber: 1.3g

Keto Avocado Smoothie

Servings: 2 | Time: 10 mins | Difficulty: Easy

INGREDIENTS:

- 1/2 Tsp. Turmeric Powder
- 1 Tsp. Fresh Ginger, Grated
- 1/4 Cup Almond Milk
- 3/4 Cup Coconut Milk
- 1/2 Avocado
- 1 Tsp. Lime Or Lemon Juice
- 1 Cup Ice, Crushed
- Stevia, To Taste

DIRECTIONS:

1. Combine all the INGREDIENTS:in a blender and blend until a smooth consistency is attained.
2. Pour in your favorite glasses and enjoy.

Nutrients per serving: Calories: 232 kcal | Fat: 22.4g | Carbohydrates: 6.9g | Protein: 1.7g | Fiber: 2.8g

Avocado Mint Green Keto Smoothie

Servings: 1 | Time: 2 mins | Difficulty: Easy

INGREDIENTS:

- ➢ 1/2 Cup Almond Milk
- ➢ 5-6 Mint Leaves
- ➢ 1/2 Avocado
- ➢ 3/4 Cup Coconut Milk
- ➢ 1/2 Tsp. Lime Juice
- ➢ 1 & 1/2 Cups Ice, Crushed
- ➢ Stevia, To Taste
- ➢ 3 Cilantro Sprigs
- ➢ 1/4 Tsp. Vanilla Extract

DIRECTIONS:

1. Combine all the INGREDIENTS:in a blender, except ice, and blend until it becomes smooth.

2. Then, add the crushed ice and blend again till the desired consistency.

3. Pour into glasses and serve.

Nutrients per serving: Calories: 223 kcal | Fat: 23g | Carbohydrates: 5g | Protein: 1g | Fiber: 1g

Keto Skinny Margaritas

Servings: 2 | Time: 10 mins | Difficulty: Easy

INGREDIENTS:

➢ 1/3 Cup Tequila

➢ 1 Tbsp. Warm Water

➢ 2 Tbsps. Lime Juice

➢ Ice Cubes, To Taste

➢ Stevia, To Taste

➢ Coarse Salt, For Glass's Rim

DIRECTIONS:

1. Mix the warm water and Stevia in a bowl and put squeeze the lime juice in another bowl.
2. Take a jar and combine the lime juice, sweetener syrup, and the tequila in it. Close the lid of the jar and shake it well to mix the contents.
3. Slightly wet the rim of two cocktail glasses and line with salt, and pour the margarita in them.
4. Add the ice in them and garnish with a slice of fresh lime if you want.

Nutrients per serving: Calories: 102 kcal | Fat: 1g | Carbohydrates: 1g | Protein: 1g

Iced Keto Matcha Green Tea Latte

Servings: 1 | Time: 1 min | Difficulty: Easy

INGREDIENTS:

➢ 5 Drops Vanilla Stevia

➢ 1 Tsp. Matcha Powder

➢ 1 Cup Coconut Or Vanilla Almond Milk, Unsweetened

➢ Ice, To Taste

DIRECTIONS:

1. Combine all ingredients:in a blender and blend for a few minutes until a smooth consistency is attained and match if completely dissolved.

2. Add ice in your preferred quantity and enjoy.

Nutrients per serving: Calories: 36 kcal | Fat: 2.5g | Carbohydrates: 0.8g | Protein: 1.6g | Fiber: 0.8g

Spiced Gingerbread Coffee

Servings: 1 | Time: 2 mins | Difficulty: Easy

INGREDIENTS:

- ➢ 1 Cup Hot Brewed Coffee
- ➢ 1 Tbsp. Heavy Cream
- ➢ 1/2 Tsp. Sukrin Gold
- ➢ 1 & 1/2 Tsps. Sukrin Gold Fiber Syrup
- ➢ 1/4 Tsp. Ginger, Ground
- ➢ 1/8 Tsp. Cloves, Ground
- ➢ 1/8 Tsp. Cinnamon, Ground
- ➢ Whipped Cream

DIRECTIONS:

1. Combine all the **INGREDIENTS:**in a mug except cloves and cream. Mix well until the spices are blended thoroughly.

2. Add a dollop of whipped cream on top and sprinkle the ground cloves on it.

Nutrients per serving: Calories: 108 kcal | Fat: 11.2g | Carbohydrates: 1.5g | Protein: 1g

Coconut Milk Strawberry Smoothie

Servings: 2 | Time: 2 mins | Difficulty: Easy

INGREDIENTS:

- ➢ 2 Tbsps. Almond Butter, Smooth
- ➢ 1 Cup Coconut Milk, Unsweetened
- ➢ 3/4 Tsp. Stevia (Optional)
- ➢ 1 Cup Strawberries, Frozen

DIRECTIONS:

1. Combine all the **INGREDIENTS:**in a blender and mix until a smooth consistency is attained.

2. Decant into the serving glasses and enjoy.

Nutrients per serving: Calories: 397 kcal | Fat: 37g | Carbohydrates: 15g | Protein: 6g | Fiber: 5g

Peanut Butter Chocolate Keto Milkshake

Servings: 1 | Time: 1 min | Difficulty: Easy

INGREDIENTS:

➢ 5 Drops Stevia

➢ 1/8 Tsp. Sea Salt

➢ 1 Tbsp. Peanut Butter Powder, Unsweetened

➢ 1 Cup Coconut Milk, Unsweetened

➢ 1 Tbsp. Cocoa Powder, Unsweetened

DIRECTIONS:

1. Combine all the INGREDIENTS:in a blender and mix until a smooth consistency is attained.

2. Decant into the serving glasses and enjoy.

Nutrients per serving: Calories: 79 kcal | Fat: 5.7g | Carbohydrates: 6.4g | Protein: 3.6g | Fiber: 3.3g

Sugar-Free Fresh Squeezed Lemonade

Servings: 8 | Time: 10 mins | Difficulty: Easy

INGREDIENTS:

- ➢ 8 Cups Water
- ➢ 1 Tsp. Lemon Monkfruit Drops
- ➢ 4 Slices Lemon (Optional)
- ➢ 3/4 Cup Lemon Juice
- ➢ Ice (Optional)

DIRECTIONS:

1. Combine all the **INGREDIENTS:**in a pitcher and stir well to mix.
2. Chill in the refrigerator or add ice to it before serving.
3. Put the lemon slices in it if you want.

Nutrients per serving: Calories: 5 kcal | Fat: 1g | Carbohydrates: 2g | Protein: 1g | Fiber: 1g

Cucumber Mint Water

Servings: 16 | Time: 5 mins | Difficulty: Easy

INGREDIENTS:

- ➢ 8 Cups Water
- ➢ 3/4 Cup Cucumber Slices
- ➢ 1 Tbsps. Mint Leaves

DIRECTIONS:

1. Press the mint leaves in a pitcher with the help of a spoon and add the other **INGREDIENTS:**to it.

2. Chill it in the refrigerator for an hour and then enjoy.

Nutrients per serving: Calories: 3 kcal | Fat: 0g | Carbohydrates: 0g | Protein: 0g | Fiber: 0g

Caramel Apple Drink

Servings: 1 | Time: 10 mins | Difficulty: Easy

INGREDIENTS:

- ➢ 2 Cups Water
- ➢ 1 Tbsp. Caramel Syrup
- ➢ 1 Tbsp. Apple Cider Vinegar (Raw)
- ➢ 1/8 Tsp. Allspice
- ➢ 1/8 Tsp. Nutmeg, Ground
- ➢ 1/8 Tsp. Orange Zest, Dried
- ➢ 1 Cinnamon Stick, Halved
- ➢ 3 Whole Cloves
- ➢ 1/4 Cup Vanilla Whipped Cream (Optional)
- ➢ 1/8 Tsp. Cinnamon, Ground (Optional)
- ➢ 5 Drops Stevia (Optional)

DIRECTIONS:

1. Take the water in a pan and put the allspice, cinnamon stick halves, and cloves in it. Boil the water and then let it sit for 2-3 minutes off the heat, with the lid on.

2. Strain the spice water into a large mug and put the caramel syrup and apple cider vinegar in it.

Stir well and add Stevia or ground cinnamon if you want.

3. Put a dollop of whipped cream on top if you ant and drizzle some caramel syrup if you want.

Nutrients per serving: Calories: 76 kcal | Fat: 3g | Carbohydrates: 16g | Protein: 1g | Fiber: 14g

Keto Frosty Chocolate Shake

Servings: 1 | Time: 10 mins | Difficulty: Easy

INGREDIENTS:

➢ 5 Tbsps. Almond Milk, Unsweetened

➢ 2 Tbsps. Cocoa Powder

➢ 1 & 1/2 Tsps. Truvia

➢ 1/8 Tsp. Vanilla Extract (Sugar-Free)

➢ 6 Tbsps. Heavy Whipping Cream

DIRECTIONS:

1. Combine all the **INGREDIENTS:**and whisk well to make a fluffy peak of cream.

2. Freeze the mixture for 20 minutes and then crack it open with a fork.

3. Chill it as per your preference and serve cold.

Nutrients per serving: Calories: 346 kcal | Fat: 36g | Carbohydrates: 8.4g | Protein: 4g | Fiber: 4g

Strawberry Avocado Smoothie

Servings: 2 | Time: 2 mins | Difficulty: Easy

INGREDIENTS:

- ➤ & 1/2 Cups Coconut Milk
- ➤ Tsp. Stevia
- ➤ Avocado
- ➤ Tbsp. Lime Juice
- ➤ 2/3 Cup Strawberries, Frozen
- ➤ 1/2 Cup Ice

DIRECTIONS:

1. Combine all the **INGREDIENTS:**in a blender and blend until a smooth consistency is attained.

2. Pour in your favorite glasses and enjoy.

Nutrients per serving: Calories: 165 kcal | Fat: 14g| Carbohydrates: 11g | Protein: 2g | Fiber: 7g

Almond Berry Mini Cheesecake Smoothies

Servings: 2 | Time: 10 mins | Difficulty: Easy

INGREDIENTS:

- ➢ 1 Cup Almond Or Coconut Milk, Chilled
- ➢ 2 Tbsps. Almond Or Coconut Flour
- ➢ 2 Cups Mixed Berries, Frozen
- ➢ 1 Tbsp. Almond Butter, Smooth
- ➢ 1/2 Cup Cottage Cheese, Organic
- ➢ 1 Tsp. Nuts Or Almonds, Toasted & Crushed
- ➢ 1 Tsp. Vanilla Extract
- ➢ 1/8 Tsp. Cinnamon
- ➢ Stevia, To Taste (Optional)

DIRECTIONS:

1. Combine all the **INGREDIENTS:**in a blender, except crushed nuts, and blend until a smooth consistency is attained.

2. You can add Stevia if you want and pour it into cups.

3. Top with crushed and toasted nuts and serve.

<u>Nutrients per serving:</u> Calories: 165 kcal | Fat: 8.6g | Carbohydrates: 16.8g | Protein: 7g | Fiber: 4.4g

Hemp Milk And Nut Milk

Servings: 4 | Time: 12 hrs. 15 mins | Difficulty: Easy

INGREDIENTS:

Nut milk

- ➢ 4 Cups Water
- ➢ 1/8 Tsp. Sea Salt
- ➢ 1 Cup Raw Nuts (Pecan, Almond, Walnut, Cashew, etc.)
- ➢ 1 Tsp. Vanilla Extract (Optional)
- ➢ 1/3 Cup Maple Syrup (Optional)

  For Hemp Milk

- ➢ 3 Cups Water
- ➢ 1/8 Tsp. Sea Salt
- ➢ 1/2 Cup Hulled Hemp Seed
- ➢ 1/4 Cup Maple Syrup (Optional)
- ➢ 1 Tsp. Vanilla Extract (Optional)

DIRECTIONS:

Nut Milk

1. Soak the nuts overnight and drain them the next day.

2. Blend the water and soaked nuts in a blender until a smooth consistency is attained.

3. Add in the salt, vanilla extract, and maple syrup if you want and blend again until mixed well.

4. Strain the mixture using a double layer of cheesecloth to isolate the pulp. Once done, add water to the milk to get your preferred consistency.

5. Pour the nut milk into mason jars and store them if you want for up to 5 days.

6. Cover the jars with lids and store in the refrigerator for up to 5 days.

Hemp Milk

1. Combine all the **INGREDIENTS:**in a blender and blend for a few minutes or until a smooth consistency is attained.

2. You can strain the excess seeds using a cheesecloth and store the hemp milk in mason jars for up to 5 days.

Gut Healing Bone Broth Latte

Servings: 2 | Time: 10 mins | Difficulty: Easy

INGREDIENTS:

➢ 1 Tbsp. Coconut Oil

➢ 1/4 Tsp. Ginger, Ground

➢ 2 Cups Bone Broth

➢ 1/8 Tsp. Cayenne Pepper

➢ 1/8 Tsp. Turmeric Powder

➢ 1/8 Tsp. Black Pepper

➢ 1/8 Tsp. Sea Salt

➢ Coconut Cream, To Taste (Optional)

➢ Collagen Peptides (Optional)

Savory Latte Toppings (Optional)

➢ Fresh Herbs

➢ Green Onion, Chopped

➢ Red Pepper Flakes

DIRECTIONS:

1. Pour bone broth into a saucepan and add all the **INGREDIENTS:**in it except sea salt.

2. Heat the mixture over medium flame while stirring constantly until combined.

3. You can use an immersion blender to mix coconut cream if necessary.
4. Blend well to make a frothy and creamy mixture.
5. Pour into serving mugs and sprinkle seal salt on top.
6. You can also use savory latte toppings for garnishing if you want.

Creamy Cocoa Coconut Low Carb Shake

Servings: 2 | Time: 5 mins | Difficulty: Easy

INGREDIENTS:

- ➢ 2 Tbsps. Cocoa Powder
- ➢ 1/2 Tbsp. Almond Butter, Smooth
- ➢ 1 Cup Almond Or Coconut Milk, Unsweetened
- ➢ 2 Tbsps. Coconut MCT Oil
- ➢ 1/8 Tsp. Sea Salt
- ➢ 1/2 Cup Coconut Cream

Additional Sweeteners (Optional)

- ➢ Stevia Leaf Or Xylitol
- ➢ Banana Or Maple Syrup
- ➢ Cinnamon
- ➢ Berries

DIRECTIONS:

1. Combine all the INGREDIENTS:in a blender and mix until a smooth consistency is attained.

2. Add sweetener of your choice, if you want, and decant into the serving glasses and enjoy.

Nutrients per serving: Calories: 222 kcal | Fat: 23.1g | Carbohydrates: 5.4g | Protein: 2.5g | Fiber: 2.7g

Low Carb Dark Chocolate Protein Smoothie

Servings: 1 | Time: 5 mins | Difficulty: Easy

INGREDIENTS:

- ➢ 1 Cup Almond Milk, Unsweetened
- ➢ 1/4 Cup Avocado, Frozen
- ➢ 1/2 Tsp. Matcha Green Tea
- ➢ 2 Tbsps. Protein Powder, Zero Carb
- ➢ 1 Tbsp. Swerve Sweetener
- ➢ 1 Tbsp. Cocoa Powder, Dark

DIRECTIONS:

1. Combine all the **INGREDIENTS:**in a blender and mix until a smooth consistency is attained.
2. Decant into the serving glass and enjoy.

Mint Chocolate Green Smoothie

Servings: 2 | Time: 5 mins | Difficulty: Easy

INGREDIENTS:

- ➤ 3/4 Cup Vanilla Almond Milk, Unsweetened
- ➤ 1/2 Cup Ice
- ➤ 1/2 Cup Kale, Packed Firmly
- ➤ 1/4 Cup Vanilla Protein Powder
- ➤ 1/4 Cup Vanilla Greek Yogurt (2%)
- ➤ 1/4 Cup Avocado, Mashed
- ➤ 1 Tbsp. Mini Chocolate Chips
- ➤ 1/4 Tsp. Peppermint Extract
- ➤ 1/2 Tbsp. Agave

DIRECTIONS:

1. Combine all the INGREDIENTS:in a blender and mix until a smooth consistency is attained.

2. Decant into the serving glasses and enjoy.

Nutrients per serving: Calories: 359 kcal | Fat: 17.4g | Carbohydrates: 37.4g | Protein: 20.6g | Fiber: 10g

Low Carb Raspberry Cheesecake Shake

Servings: 1 | Time: 5 mins | Difficulty: Easy

INGREDIENTS:

➢ 1/4 Cup Almond Milk, Unsweetened

➢ 1 Tsp. Butter, Unsalted (Cold)

➢ 1/4 Cup Heavy Cream

➢ 6-8 Raspberries, Fresh

➢ 1/4 Cup Cream Cheese

➢ 4 Tsps. Almond Flour

➢ Ice (Optional)

➢ Liquid Stevia, To Taste (Optional)

DIRECTIONS:

1. Put the almond milk, raspberries, heavy cream, and cream cheese in a vessel and blend using an immersion blender. Add the sweetener if you want. Transfer it into a serving glass.

2. In a bowl, mix the almond flour and butter to form crumbs. Put these crumbs on top of the drink after adding ice, if you want, and serve.

Nutrients per serving: Calories: 560 kcal | Fat: 55g | Carbohydrates: 8g | Protein: 9g | Fiber: 3g

Watermelon Smoothie

Servings: 1 | Time: 5 mins | Difficulty: Easy

INGREDIENTS:

- 3/4 Cup Lemon Lime Seltzer
- 1/8 Tsp. Xantham Gum
- 15 Drops Watermelon Flavoring Oil
- 8 Ice Cubes
- 1 Drop Vanilla Extract
- 2 Tbsps. Stevia
- 1 Drop Lemon Extract
- 1. Tbsp Heavy Cream

DIRECTIONS:

1. Combine all the INGREDIENTS:in a blender and mix until a smooth consistency is attained.
2. Decant into the serving glass and enjoy.

Nutrients per serving: Calories: 39 kcal | Fat: 3g | Carbohydrates: 1g | Protein: 0g

Low-Carb Blueberry Smoothie

Servings: 2 | Time: 5 mins | Difficulty: Easy

INGREDIENTS:

- ➢ 1/4 Cup Cream Cheese
- ➢ 3/4 Cup Almond Milk, Unsweetened
- ➢ 1/2 Tsp. Vanilla Extract
- ➢ 1/2 Cup Ice
- ➢ 2 Tsps. Stevia/Erythritol Blend, Granulated
- ➢ 1/3 Cup Blueberries, Frozen
- ➢ 1-5 Drops Lemon Extract
- ➢ 1/4 Cup Heavy Whipping Cream
- ➢ 2 Tbsps. Collagen Peptides (Optional)

DIRECTIONS:

1. Combine all the INGREDIENTS:in a blender and mix until a smooth consistency is attained.

2. Decant into the serving glasses and enjoy.

Nutrients per serving: Calories: 251 kcal | Fat: 22g | Carbohydrates: 6g | Protein: 8g | Fiber: 1g

Pumpkin Low Carb Smoothie With Salted Caramel

Servings: 1 | Time: 5 mins | Difficulty: Easy

INGREDIENTS:

- ➢ 1 Cup Almond Milk
- ➢ 1/4 Avocado
- ➢ 2 Tbsps. Vanilla Protein Powder
- ➢ 1/4 Cup Pumpkin Puree
- ➢ 4 Ice Cubes
- ➢ 2 Tbsps. Caramel Syrup, Salted & Sugar-Free

DIRECTIONS:

1. Combine all the **INGREDIENTS:**in a blender and mix until a smooth consistency is attained.

2. Decant into the serving glass and enjoy.

Nutrients per serving: Calories: 245 kcal | Fat: 10.4g | Carbohydrates: 11.8g | Protein: 29g | Fiber: 6.4g

McKeto Strawberry Milkshake

Servings: 1 | Time: 5 mins | Difficulty: Easy

INGREDIENTS:

- ➢ 1/4 Cup Heavy Cream
- ➢ 1/4 Tsp. Xanthan Gum
- ➢ 3/4 Cup Coconut Milk
- ➢ 7 Ice Cubes
- ➢ 1 Tbsp. MCT Oil
- ➢ 2 Tbsps. Strawberry Torani, Sugar-Free

DIRECTIONS:

1. Combine all the **INGREDIENTS:**in a blender and mix until a smooth consistency is attained.

2. Decant into the serving glass and enjoy.

Nutrients per serving: Calories: 368 kcal | Fat: 38.85g | Carbohydrates: 2.42g | Protein: 1.69g | Fiber: 1.28g

Keto Blueberry Cheesecake Smoothie

Servings: 1 | Time: 5 mins | Difficulty: Easy

INGREDIENTS:

- 1/2 Cup Cream Cheese
- 2 Tbsps. Heavy Cream
- 1 Cup Almond Milk, Unsweetened
- 1 Tsp. Cinnamon, Ground
- 1/2 Cup Blueberries
- 6 Drops Stevia
- 1/2 Tsp. Vanilla Extract

DIRECTIONS:

1. Combine all the INGREDIENTS:in a blender and mix until a smooth consistency is attained.
2. Decant into the serving glass and enjoy.

Nutrients per serving: Calories: 311 kcal | Fat: 27g | Carbohydrates: 9g | Protein: 5.5g | Fiber: 2.5g

Keto Tropical Smoothie

Servings: 2 | Time: 5 mins | Difficulty: Easy

INGREDIENTS:

- ➢ 1 Tbsp. MCT Oil
- ➢ 1/2 Tsp. Mango Extract
- ➢ 7 Ice Cubes
- ➢ 2 Tbsps. Golden Flaxseed Meal
- ➢ 1/4 Tsp. Blueberry Extract
- ➢ 3/4 Cup Coconut Milk, Unsweetened
- ➢ 1/4 Tsp. Banana Extract
- ➢ 1/4 Cup Sour Cream
- ➢ 20 Drops Liquid Stevia

DIRECTIONS:

- Combine all the **INGREDIENTS:**in a blender and mix until a smooth consistency is attained. Let it sit for a few minutes and allow the flax meal to absorb moisture.

- Decant into the serving glasses and enjoy.

Nutrients per serving: Calories: 355.75 kcal | Fat: 32.63g | Carbohydrates: 4.41g | Protein: 4.4g | Fiber: 3g

Keto Kale & Coconut Shake

Servings: 1 | Time: 5 mins | Difficulty: Easy

INGREDIENTS:

- ➢ 4 Cups Kale, Chopped
- ➢ 1/2 Cup Coconut Milk
- ➢ 1 Cup Almond Milk, Unsweetened
- ➢ 1/4 Cup Coconut, Unsweetened & Ground
- ➢ 1 Cup Ice
- ➢ 1/4 Tsp. Kosher Salt
- ➢ 1 Tbsp. Fresh Ginger, Peeled (Optional)

DIRECTIONS:

1. Combine all the **INGREDIENTS:**in a blender and mix until a smooth consistency is attained.
2. Decant into the serving glass and enjoy.

Nutrients per serving: Calories: 660 kcal | Fat: 60g | Carbohydrates: 7g | Protein: 13g | Fiber: 7g

Savory Cucumber Herb Sangria

Servings: 2-4 | Time: 5 mins | Difficulty: Easy

INGREDIENTS:

- 2 Cups Sparkling Water
- 3 Cups Dry White Wine
- 2 Cups Ice
- 3 Limes, Sliced
- 1 Green Cucumber, Sliced
- 1 Cup Basil Leaves, Fresh
- 2 Lemons, Sliced
- 1 Cup Mint Leaves, Fresh

DIRECTIONS:

- Put all **INGREDIENTS:**in a pitcher except wine, sparkling water, and ice. Stir well and press the lemon, lime, basil, mint, and cucumber a little to release their juices.
- Add the wine to it and stir well.
- Put it in the refrigerator and let it sit for about 20 minutes.
- Take out the pitcher and pour in the sparkling water and ice.

➢ Serve cold.

<u>Nutrients per serving:</u> Calories: 660 kcal | Fat: 60g | Carbohydrates: 7g | Protein: 13g | Fiber: 7g

Sparkling Raspberry Limeade Mocktail

Servings: 2 | Time: 1 min | Difficulty: Easy

INGREDIENTS:

➢ 1/2 Cup Raspberries, Unsweetened & Frozen

➢ 1 & 1/2 Cups Sparkling Raspberry Lemonade, Chilled

➢ 2 Tbsps. Lime Juice

➢ 1/8 Tsp. Vanilla Stevia

➢ 1/2 Cup Ice, Crushed

DIRECTIONS:

1. Combine all the **INGREDIENTS:**in a blender and mix until a smooth consistency is attained.

2. Decant into the serving glasses and enjoy.

Nutrients per serving: Calories: 22 kcal | Fat: 0.2g | Carbohydrates: 5.5g | Protein: 0.5g | Fiber: 2.1g

Bailey's Irish Cream

Servings: 12 | Time: 20 mins | Difficulty: Easy

INGREDIENTS:

➢ 1/2 Tsp. Vanilla Extract

➢ 1 & 1/4 Cups Irish Whiskey

➢ 2 Cups Heavy Cream

➢ 1 Tbsp. Cocoa Powder

➢ 1/2 Tsp. Instant Espresso Powder

➢ 2/3 Cup Swerve

➢ 1 Tsp. Almond Extract

DIRECTIONS:

1. Take a saucepan and put cocoa, instant powder, sweetener, and cream in it. Heat it over medium-low flame and bring to a boil.

2. Reduce heat to low and let it simmer for about 10 minutes.

3. Take off the heat and add in the whiskey, almond, and vanilla extracts.

4. Let cool and serve.

Nutrients per serving: Calories: 200 kcal | Fat: 14g | Carbohydrates: 1g | Protein: 0g | Fiber: 0g

Low Carb Coffee Milkshake

Servings: 2 | Time: 1 min | Difficulty: Easy

INGREDIENTS:

- ➢ 1 Tsp. Instant Espresso Powder

- ➢ 15 Drops Stevia

- ➢ 1 & 1/2 Cups Ice, Crushed

- ➢ 1 Cup Vanilla Ice Cream (Low Carb)

- ➢ 1/2 Cup Almond Milk

- ➢ 2 Tsps. Cocoa Powder (Optional)

- ➢ 2 Tbsps. Whipped Cream (Optional)

DIRECTIONS:

1. Combine all the **INGREDIENTS:**in a blender and mix until a smooth consistency is attained.

2. Decant into the serving glasses and put a dollop of whipped cream on top if you want.

Nutrients per serving: Calories: 345 kcal | Fat: 31.4g | Carbohydrates: 24g | Protein: 2.5g | Fiber: 18.2g

Sugar-Free Strawberry Limeade

Servings: 8 | Time: 5 mins | Difficulty: Easy

INGREDIENTS:

- ➢ 5 Cups Water

- ➢ 3/4 Cup Lime Juice, Fresh

- ➢ 1 & 1/2 Tsps. Stevia

- ➢ 1 & 1/2 Cups Strawberries, Sliced

- ➢ Ice, To Taste

DIRECTIONS:

1. Combine all the **INGREDIENTS:**in a blender and mix until a smooth consistency is attained.

2. Decant into the serving glasses and enjoy.

Nutrients per serving: Calories: 16 kcal | Fat: 0.1g | Carbohydrates: 4.3g | Protein: 0.2g | Fiber: 1.5g

Low-Carb Keto Shamrock Shake

Servings: 1 | Time: 2 mins | Difficulty: Easy

INGREDIENTS:

- ➤ 1 Tsp. Spinach Powder
- ➤ 1 Cup Vanilla Ice Cream, Low Carb
- ➤ 1/3 Cup Coconut Or Almond Milk, Unsweetened
- ➤ 1/8 Tsp. Pure Mint Extract
- ➤ Whipped Cream (Optional)

DIRECTIONS:

- Combine all the **INGREDIENTS:**in a blender and mix until a smooth consistency is attained.
- Decant into the serving glasses and put a dollop of whipped cream on top if you want.

Keto Smoothie With Almond Milk

Servings: 1 | Time: 5 mins | Difficulty: Easy

INGREDIENTS:

- ➢ 1 Tbsp. Cocoa Powder, Unsweetened
- ➢ 2 Tbsps. Almond Butter
- ➢ 1 Cup Almond Milk
- ➢ 1/4 Cup Avocado
- ➢ 3 Tbsps. Monkfruit
- ➢ 1 Cup Ice, Crushed

DIRECTIONS:

1. Combine all the INGREDIENTS:in a blender and mix until a smooth consistency is attained.

2. Decant into the serving glass and enjoy.

Nutrients per serving: Calories: 332 kcal | Fat: 28.5g | Carbohydrates: 15g | Protein: 10.2g | Fiber: 8.9g

Sparkling Grapefruit Frosé

Servings: 6 | Time: 5 mins | Difficulty: Easy

INGREDIENTS:

➢ 1 Cup Ice

➢ 1 Cup Grapefruit Juice, Fresh

➢ 1/4 Cup Agave Nectar

➢ 1 & 1/2 Cups Rosé Wine

For Garnish (Optional)

➢ Grapefruit Wedges

➢ Mint Sprigs

DIRECTIONS:

1. Freeze rosé in a shallow dish overnight.

2. Scrape it off the dish the next day and put in a blender with all other ingredients.

3. Blend until a smooth consistency is attained.

4. Decant into the serving glasses and garnish with mint sprigs and grapefruit wedges if you want.

Nutrients per serving: Calories: 244 kcal | Fat: 0.1g | Carbohydrates: 29.1g | Protein: 1g | Fiber: 0.1g

Banana Oat Breakfast Smoothie

Servings: 2 | Time: 5 mins | Difficulty: Easy

INGREDIENTS:

➢ 1 Banana

➢ 1/2 Cup Almond Milk

➢ 1 Tbsp. Flaxseed Meal

➢ 1/2 Cup Yogurt

➢ 1/2 Tsp. Cinnamon

➢ 1/3 Cup Rolled Oats

DIRECTIONS:

1. Combine all the INGREDIENTS:in a blender and mix until a smooth consistency is attained.

2. Decant into the serving glasses and enjoy.

Nutrients per serving: Calories: 210 kcal | Fat: 7.5g | Carbohydrates: 32.5g | Protein: 5.6g | Fiber: 4.8g

Keto Mexican Chocolate Eggnog

Servings: 6 | Time: 15 mins | Difficulty: Easy

INGREDIENTS:

- ➢ 1/4 Cup Whiskey Or Bourbon
- ➢ 1 & 1/2 Cups Almond Milk, Unsweetened
- ➢ 6 Eggs
- ➢ 1/4 Cup Cocoa Powder
- ➢ 1/2 Cup Monkfruit/Erythritol Blend
- ➢ 1 Cup Heavy Cream
- ➢ 1/2 Cup Whipped Cream
- ➢ 1 Tsp. Vanilla
- ➢ 1/2 Tsp. Cinnamon Powder
- ➢ 1/4 Tsp. Chili Powder
- ➢ 1/8 Tsp. Cayenne Pepper
- ➢ 1/8 Tsp. Nutmeg, Grated
- ➢ 1/8 Tsp. Salt

DIRECTIONS:

1. Combine all the **INGREDIENTS:**in a blender except bourbon/whiskey, vanilla, and whipped cream. Blend it until a smooth consistency is attained.

2. Then pour this mixture into a saucepan and heat it over a medium-low flame with constant stirring for about 8 minutes. Do not let it boil.

3. Take off the heat, put the saucepan in a bowl full of ice, and stir the eggnog to cool it down.

4. Add the bourbon/whiskey and vanilla in it and decant into a covered container.

5. Refrigerate for about 4 hours and add in the whipped cream or top the eggnog with it.

6. Serve and enjoy.

Nutrients per serving: Calories: 242 kcal | Fat: 23g | Carbohydrates: 4g | Protein: 7g | Fiber: 1g

Keto Cranberry Hibiscus Margarita

Servings: 8 | Time: 20 mins | Difficulty: Easy

INGREDIENTS:

- ➢ 2 & 1/2 Tbsps. Naval Orange Zest
- ➢ 1 & 1/2 Cups Cranberries, Fresh Cup Tequila
- ➢ 5 Cup Water
- ➢ 3/4 Cups + 2 Tbsps. Monkfruit/Erythritol Blend
- ➢ 1 Tbsps. Lime Juice, Fresh
- ➢ Ice
- ➢ Hibiscus Tea Bags
- ➢ Coarse Salt, For Glass's Rim

DIRECTIONS:

1. Take a saucepan and put the 1 cup water, 3/4 cup sweetener, orange zest, and cranberries in it. Heat it over medium flame and bring to boil, reduce heat, and let it simmer until it is thickened, for about 10-15 minutes.

2. Strain the cranberry gel and let cool.

3. Boil the remaining 4 cups of water in a saucepan and put the hibiscus tea bags in it for five minutes.

4. Take out the tea bags and add the 2 Tbsps. of sweetener in it. Mix well and set aside to cool down.

5. Combine the cranberry gel, hibiscus tea, and all the remaining ingredients_in a blender and blend well.

6. Slightly wet the rim of cocktail glasses and line with salt, and pour the margarita in them.

Nutrients per serving: Calories: 86 kcal | Fat: 1g | Carbohydrates: 6g | Protein: 1g | Fiber: 2g

Keto Frozen Blackberry Lemonade

Servings: 2 | Time: 5 mins | Difficulty: Easy

INGREDIENTS:

➢ 1 Cup Ice

➢ 1/4 Cup Blackberries, Fresh

➢ 4 Tbsps. Lemon Juice

➢ 1/2 Cup Almond Milk

➢ 1/3 Cup Coconut Cream

➢ 1 Tbsp. Stevia/Erythritol Blend

➢ 1/8 Tsp. Sea Salt

DIRECTIONS:

1. Combine all the ingrediente in a blender and mix until a smooth consistency is attained.

2. Decant into the serving glasses and enjoy.

Nutrients per serving: Calories: 155 kcal | Fat: 15g | Carbohydrates: 6g | Protein: 2g | Fiber: 2g

Triple Berry Cheesecake Smoothie

Servings: 1 | Time: 5 mins | Difficulty: Easy

INGREDIENTS:

- ➢ 2 Tbsps. Avocado

- ➢ 1/2 Cup Mixed Berries, Frozen

- ➢ 1 Tsp. Vanilla

- ➢ 2 Tbsps. Cream Cheese

- ➢ 1/8 Tsp. Sea Salt

- ➢ 1/2 Cup Almond Milk, Unsweetened

- ➢ 7-10 Drops Monkfruit Extract

DIRECTIONS:

1. Combine all the ingredients in a blender and mix until a smooth consistency is attained.

2. Decant into the serving glass and enjoy.

Nutrients per serving: Calories: 158 kcal | Fat: 11g | Carbohydrates: 12g | Protein: 3g | Fiber: 6g

ServMaple Almond

servings: 1 | Time: 5 mins | Difficulty: Easy

INGREDIENTS:

- ➢ 1 Cup Baby Spinach
- ➢ 1 Tbsp. Avocado
- ➢ 1 Tbsp. Golden Flax Meal
- ➢ 1 Tbsp. Almond Butter
- ➢ 1 Cup Almond Milk, Unsweetened
- ➢ 1 & 1/4 Tsps. Stevia/Erythritol Blend
- ➢ 1/4 Tsp. Vanilla Extract
- ➢ 1/8 Tsp. Cinnamon
- ➢ 1/4 Tsp. Maple Extract
- ➢ 2-3 Ice Cubes (Optional)

DIRECTIONS:

1. Combine all the ingredient in a blender and mix until a smooth consistency is attained.

2. Decant into the serving glass and enjoy.

Nutrients per serving: Calories: 210 kcal | Fat: 16.8g | Carbohydrates: 10.4g | Protein: 8.1g | Fiber: 6.3g

Dairy Free Chocolate Pecan Keto Shake

Servings: 1 | Time: 10 mins | Difficulty: Easy

INGREDIENTS:

- ➤ 5 Raw Pecans, Halved
- ➤ 2 Tbsps. Cocoa Powder, Unsweetened
- ➤ 1/8 Tsp. Pink Himalayan Salt
- ➤ 1 & 1/3 Cups Almond Milk, Unsweetened
- ➤ 1 & 1/2 Tsps. Stevia/Erythritol Blend
- ➤ 1 Tbsps. Avocado
- ➤ 3-4 Ice Cubes

DIRECTIONS:

1. Combine all the ingredients in a blender and mix until a smooth consistency is attained.

2. Decant into the serving glass and enjoy.

Nutrients per serving: Calories: 247 kcal | Fat: 20g | Carbohydrates: 12g | Protein: 5g | Fiber: 8g

Strawberry Colada Milkshake

Servings: 1 | Time: 3 mins | Difficulty: Easy

INGREDIENTS:

- 1/2 Tbsp. Chia Seeds
- 3-4 Strawberries, Frozen
- 1/3 Cup Coconut Milk
- 1/3 Cup Almond Milk, Unsweetened
- 1 Tsp. Stevia/Erythritol Blend
- 4-5 Ice Cubes
- 1/8 Tsp. Pink Salt
- 1/4 Tsp. Coconut Extract
- 1/4 Tsp. Vanilla Extract
- 1/2 Tbsp. Coconut Oil (Optional)
- 1 Tbsp. Strawberries, Freeze-Dried (Optional)

DIRECTIONS:

1. Combine all the ingredients in a blender and mix until a smooth consistency is attained.

2. Decant into the serving glass and enjoy.

Nutrients per serving: Calories: 660 kcal | Fat: 60g | Carbohydrates: 7g | Protein: 13g | Fiber: 7g

Keto Frozen Hot Chocolate

Servings: 1 | Time: 5 mins | Difficulty: Easy

INGREDIENTS:

- ➤ 1 Tbsp. Avocado
- ➤ 1/4 Cup Coconut Milk
- ➤ 1 Tbsp. Cocoa
- ➤ 1/2 Cup Almond Milk, Unsweetened
- ➤ 1/2 Cup Ice Cubes
- ➤ 1 & 1/4 Tsps. Stevia/Erythritol Blend
- ➤ 1/2 Tsp. Vanilla
- ➤ 1/8 Tsp. Pink Himalayan Salt

For Garnish

- ➤ Chocolate Chips, Sugar-Free
- ➤ Whipped Coconut Cream

DIRECTIONS:

1. Combine all the ingredients in a blender except ice cubes. Blend until a smooth consistency is attained.

2. Decant into the serving glass, add the ice, and put the whipped cream and chocolate chips on top if you want.

<u>Nutrients per serving:</u> Calories: 660 kcal | Fat: 60g | Carbohydrates: 7g | Protein: 13g | Fiber: 7g

Dairy-Free Keto Iced Latte

Servings: 1 | Time: 5 mins | Difficulty: Easy

INGREDIENTS:

➢ 1/4 Cup Brewed Coffee, Strong

➢ 1 & 1/2 Cups Almond Milk, Unsweetened

➢ 1 Tbsp. MCT Oil

DIRECTIONS:

1. Brew your coffee according to your preference.

2. Combine all the ingredients in a blender and mix until a smooth consistency is attained.

3. Decant into the serving cup and enjoy.

Nutrients per serving: Calories: 660 kcal | Fat: 60g | Carbohydrates: 7g | Protein: 13g | Fiber: 7g

Sugar-Free Hibiscus Lemonade

Servings: 4 | Time: 10 mins | Difficulty: Easy

INGREDIENTS:

➢ 1 & 1/2 Cups Sparkling Mineral Water

➢ 2 Tbsps. Lemon Juice, Fresh

➢ 1 Tbsp. Stevia/Erythritol Blend

➢ 2 Cups Brewed Hibiscus Tea

➢ Ice, To Taste

DIRECTIONS:

1. Put all the ingredients in a pitcher except water and ice. Mix everything well until dissolved.

2. Add the water and ice and stir.

3. Decant into the serving glasses and enjoy.

Nutrients per serving: Calories: 660 kcal | Fat: 60g | Carbohydrates: 7g | Protein: 13g | Fiber: 7g

Low Carb 7Up

Servings: 2 | Time: 2 mins | Difficulty: Easy

INGREDIENTS:

- ➢ 1 & 1/2 Cups Ice
- ➢ 1/4 Tsp. Liquid Stevia
- ➢ 1/2 Tbsp. Lime Juice
- ➢ 2/3 Cup Seltzer Water

DIRECTIONS:

1. Fill serving glass with ice and put all the other ingredients in it.

2. Stir well and enjoy.

Nutrients per serving: Calories: 2 kcal | Fat: 0g | Carbohydrates: 1g | Protein: 0g | Fiber: 0g

Low Carb German Chocolate Fat Bomb Hot Chocolate

Servings: 1 | Time: 12 mins | Difficulty: Easy

INGREDIENTS:

➢ 2 Tbsps. Cocoa Butter

➢ 1/4 Cup Coconut Milk

➢ 1 Cup Chocolate Almond Milk, Unsweetened

➢ Stevia, To Taste

DIRECTIONS:

1. In a saucepan, combine all the ingredients and heat over medium-low flame until the cocoa butter melts.

2. Remove from the heat and mix with an immersion blender till t becomes frothy.

3. Decant into your favorite mug and enjoy.

Nutrients per serving: Calories: 358 kcal | Fat: 39g | Carbohydrates: 2g | Protein: 2g

Low Carb German Gingerbread Hot Chocolate

Servings: 2 | Time: 20 mins | Difficulty: Easy

INGREDIENTS:

➢ 1/4 Cup Cocoa Powder, Unsweetened

➢ 2 Cups Chocolate Almond Milk, Unsweetened

➢ 1/2 Tsp. Liquid Stevia

➢ 1/4 Cup Stevia

➢ 1/4 Tsp. Cardamom, Ground

➢ 1 Tsp. Cinnamon, Ground

➢ 1/8 Tsp. Allspice, Ground

➢ 1/8 Tsp. Anise Seed, Ground

➢ 1/8 Tsp. Cloves, Ground

➢ 1/8 Tsp. Nutmeg, Ground

➢ 1/8 Tsp. Ginger, Ground

DIRECTIONS:

1. Combine all the ingredients in a saucepan and heat it over medium heat.

2. Once it boils, reduce the heat to low, and let it simmer for about 5 minutes with intermittent stirring.

3. Decant into serving mugs and enjoy.

Nutrients per serving: Calories: 72 kcal | Fat: 4g | Carbohydrates: 11g | Protein: 3g | Fiber: 5g

Coconut Pumpkin Steamer

Servings: 1 | Time: 5 mins | Difficulty: Easy

INGREDIENTS:

- ➢ 1 Tsp. Vanilla Extract
- ➢ 1/2 Cup Coconut Milk
- ➢ Stevia, To Taste
- ➢ 1/4 Tsp. Pumpkin Pie Spice, Without Sugar

DIRECTIONS:

1. Combine all the ingredients in a saucepan and heat it over medium heat.

2. Once the bubbles start to form, take off the heat, and serve warm.

Nutrients per serving: Calories: 241 kcal | Fat: 24g | Carbohydrates: 9g | Protein: 2g | Fiber: 1g

Low Carb Margarita Mix

Servings: 2 | Time: 5 mins | Difficulty: Easy

INGREDIENTS:

- ➤ 1/2 Cup Lemon Juice, Fresh
- ➤ 1 & 1/2 Cups Water
- ➤ 1/4 Tsp. Liquid Stevia
- ➤ 1/3 Cup Erythritol, Powdered
- ➤ 1/8 Tsp. Orange Extract
- ➤ 1 Cup Tequila
- ➤ Ice, To Taste

DIRECTIONS:

1. Combine all the ingredients in a pitcher except tequila and ice.

2. Mix well to dissolve the sweetener.

3. Add the tequila and stir.

4. Pour in the cocktail glasses with rims covered with salt.

5. Add the ice and enjoy.

Nutrients per serving: Calories: 35 kcal | Fat: 0g | Carbohydrates: 9g | Protein: 0g | Fiber: 0g

Low Carb Electrolyte Water

Servings: 4 | Time: 5 mins | Difficulty: Easy

INGREDIENTS:

➢ 4 Cups Water

➢ 2 Tbsps. Lemon Juice

➢ 1/8 Tsp. Baking Soda

➢ Stevia, To Taste

➢ 1/8 Tsp. Salt

DIRECTIONS:

1. Combine all the in a bottle, cover it, and shake well.

2. Serve and enjoy.

Nutrients per serving: Calories: 2 kcal | Fat: 0g | Carbohydrates: 1g | Protein: 0g

Low Carb Pumpkin Spice Mocha

Servings: 2 | Time: 15 mins | Difficulty: Easy

INGREDIENTS:

➢ 1 Tsp. Pumpkin Pie Spice, Without Sugar

➢ Stevia, To Taste

➢ 3 Tbsps. Cocoa Butter

➢ 1/4 Cup Coffee Grounds

➢ 3 Cups Water

DIRECTIONS:

1. Brew the coffee according to your preference with the pumpkin spice in it.

2. Add the cocoa butter in it and blend with an immersion blender until a smooth consistency is attained and it becomes frothy.

3. Add the desired quantity of sweetener and enjoy.

Nutrients per serving: Calories: 187 kcal | Fat: 21g | Carbohydrates: 1g | Protein: 0g

Kombucha Sangria

Servings: 7 | Time: 10 mins | Difficulty: Easy

INGREDIENTS:

➢ 4 Tbsps. Monkfruit, Powdered

➢ 1 Cup Orange Juice

➢ 2 Cups Kombucha

➢ 3 & 1/4 Cups Spanish Wine

➢ 1 Lime, Sliced

➢ 1 Orange, Sliced

➢ 1 Lemon, Sliced

➢ 1/2 Cup Brandy (Optional)

DIRECTIONS:

1. Combine all the ingredients in a pitcher, except orange, lemon, and lime slices.

2. Stir well to mix and add the orange, lemon, and lime slices.

3. Serve with ice and enjoy.

Nutrients per serving: Calories: 101 kcal | Fat: 0g | Carbohydrates: 6.5g | Protein: 0.1g | Fiber: 0g

Pumpkin Spice Hot Buttered Rum

Servings: 4 | Time: 10 mins | Difficulty: Easy

INGREDIENTS:

➢ 1 Cup Butter

➢ 1 Cup Golden Monkfruit

➢ 3 Tbsps. Maple Syrup, Sugar-Free

➢ 2 Tsps. Vanilla Extract

➢ 1 Cup Heavy Cream

➢ 1 & 1/2 Cups Monkfruit, Powdered

➢ 1 Tbsp. Pumpkin Pie Spice

➢ 2 Cups Hot Water

➢ 1 Cup Rum

DIRECTIONS:

1. Take a bowl and put the golden Monkfruit, butter, vanilla, and maple syrup in it. Whisk well for few minutes until creamy and fluffy.

2. Add all the other ingredients except rum and water and mix well. Set aside.

3. Fill each serving glass with 1/4 cup Rum, 1/2 cup water, and two to three tbsps. of the batter and stir well.

<u>Nutrients per serving:</u> Calories: 73 kcal | Fat: 60g | Carbohydrates: 1.2g | Protein: 0.2g | Fiber: 0.5g

Tart Cherry Lemon Drop

Servings: 1 | Time: 5 mins | Difficulty: Easy

INGREDIENTS:

- ➤ 4 Tbsps. Tart Cherry Juice
- ➤ 4 Lemon Wedges
- ➤ 2 Tbsps. Fresh Lemon Juice
- ➤ 3 Tbsps. Vodka
- ➤ 2 Tbsps. Water
- ➤ 1 Tbsp. Monkfruit, Powdered
- ➤ 1 Tbsp. Lemon Juice, Fresh
- ➤ 1 Tsp. Monkfruit, Granular
- ➤ Ice, To Taste

DIRECTIONS:

1. Combine powdered lemon juice, water, and lemon wedges in a blender and blend well until a smooth consistency is attained.

2. Add the vodka, tart cherry juice, and ice in it and blend again until desires consistency.

3. Dip the rim of the cocktail glass in lemon juice and then in granular Monkfruit.

4. Pour in the juice and garnish with a lemon slice if you want.

Nutrients per serving: Calories: 660 kcal | Fat: 60g | Carbohydrates: 7g | Protein: 13g | Fiber: 7g

Orange Creamsicle Mimosas

Servings: 1 | Time: 10 mins | Difficulty: Easy

INGREDIENTS:

➢ 1 Tbsp. Vanilla Vodka

➢ 1/4 Cup Orange Juice, Fresh

➢ 2 Tbsps. Heavy Cream

➢ 1 Tsp. Monkfruit, Powdered

➢ 1/2 Cup Sparkling Wine, Dry (Prosecco Or Champagne)

DIRECTIONS:

1. Combine all the ingredients in a blender except wine. Blend it well until a smooth consistency is attained.

2. Add the wine and serve.

Nutrients per serving: Calories: 255 kcal | Fat: 11.5g | Carbohydrates: 8g | Protein: 0.9g | Fiber: 0.1g

CPSIA information can be obtained
at www.ICGtesting.com
Printed in the USA
LVHW022121110521
687091LV00012B/2415